ADDRESSING COMMON CONCERNS

Nutrition Solutions for Gestational Diabetes, Nausea, and Swelling

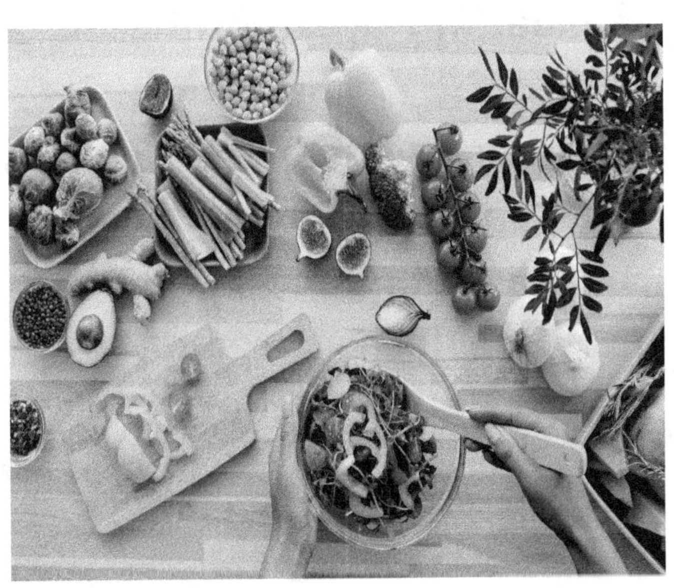

Jessica Cole

Copyright © 2023 Jessica Cole

Table of Contents

Addressing Common Concerns

Nutrition Solutions for Gestational Diabetes, Nausea, and Swelling

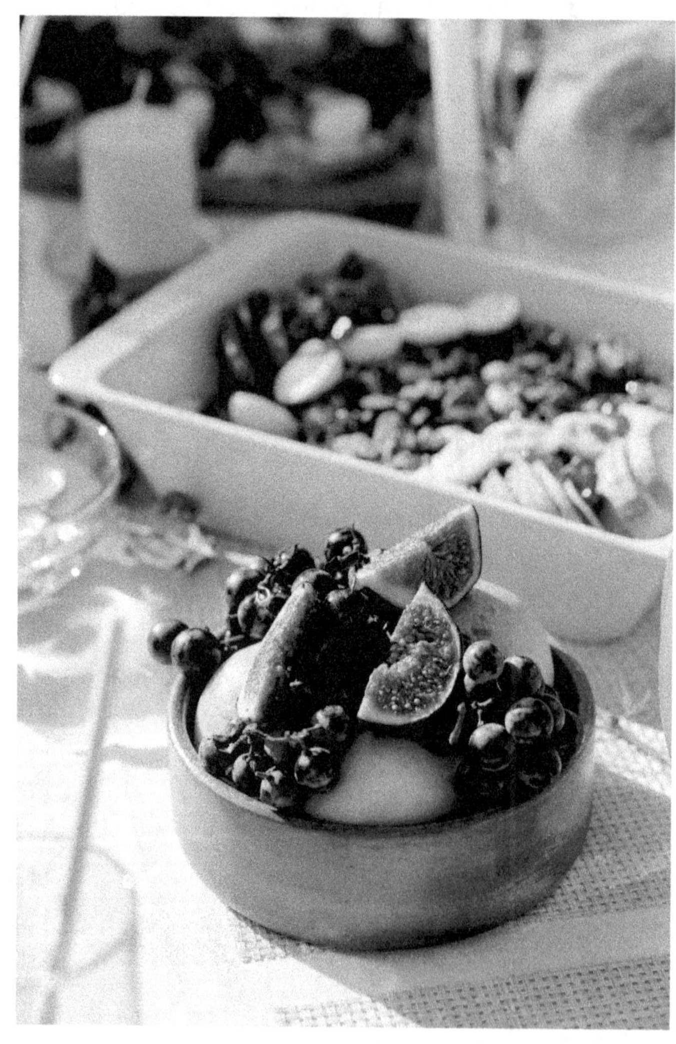

Introduction

Hello, courageous mothers on the high seas! Welcome to a voyage of care, nourishment, and empowerment as we set sail through the pages of "Addressing Common Concerns: Nutrition Solutions for Gestational Diabetes, Nausea, and Swelling." Within these chapters, we set sail to navigate the seas of pregnancy, providing guidance and support to address some of the common challenges faced during this transformative period.

While being pregnant is a time of wonder, excitement, and unending joy, it also comes with certain worries and unknowns. We find ourselves navigating through the complexities of gestational diabetes, the stormy waves of nausea, and the ebb and flow of swelling as the wind whispers through the sails of life. But do not worry, comrades, for we have the compass of knowledge and the treasure of dietary solutions at our disposal to lead us on this magnificent journey.

As we set sail across the seas of blood sugar management and the power of nutrition to guide us toward a healthy and bright pregnancy, our adventure begins with unraveling the mystery of gestational diabetes. We will create individualized food plans along the way to nourish the mother and the unborn child, guaranteeing a smooth and secure journey during pregnancy.

As we continue to sail, we run into waves of pregnant sickness, a frequent issue that can provide difficulties for even the most seasoned sailors. We'll learn about dietary techniques to relieve discomfort, making this portion of the journey easier and more pleasant for both mother and pregnancy

Pregnancy tides also cause swelling and fluid retention, which can occasionally resemble stormy seas. But don't worry; we'll look into nutrition strategies that can aid to lessen edema and help us overcome these obstacles with poise and resiliency.

We shall ground ourselves in the strength of pregnant superfoods as the chapters develop and explore the depths of nutrient-rich riches that enliven our bodies and spirits. We will strengthen our trip with these diets to ensure a plentiful and nourished pregnancy.

However, our journey goes beyond only nutrition. As we navigate the physical activity that supports gestational diabetes control, reduces nausea, and improves general well-being, we will appreciate the synergy of exercise and nutrition.

We will develop the ability to deal with food aversions and cravings in the face of constantly shifting winds, guiding our ship toward better options while respecting our desires with awareness and balance.

We become aware of the value of good hydration when we travel since it keeps us energized and fed, making every part of the trip more enjoyable and fulfilling.

We realize the value of support and self-care as we navigate the waters of pregnancy. We are aware of how crucial it is to seek expert advice, care for one's emotional well-being, and establish a thorough self-care regimen to have a happy and successful pregnancy.

Dear travelers, each chapter in these pages is a call to embrace the pregnant journey with grace and empowerment. Join us as we address common worries, appreciate the power of nutrition, and set off on a journey that celebrates the marvels of motherhood. We ask you to join us on this journey of care and discovery.

Let's raise our sails and set off on this life-changing journey together. As we navigate the waters of pregnancy with kindness, knowledge, and the nourishing power of nourishment, fair winds to you, courageous navigators. May this book serve as a beacon for you as you travel through the exquisite tapestry of pregnancy and parenting. Happy travels!

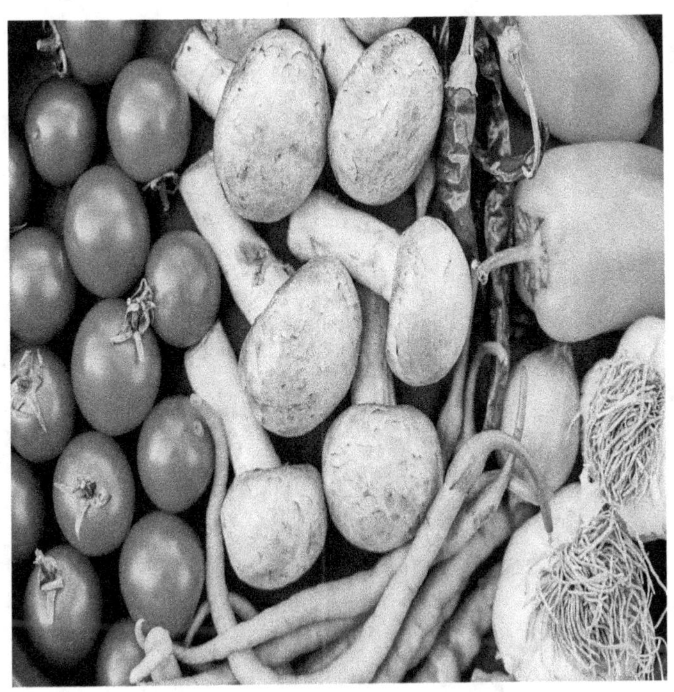

Swelling

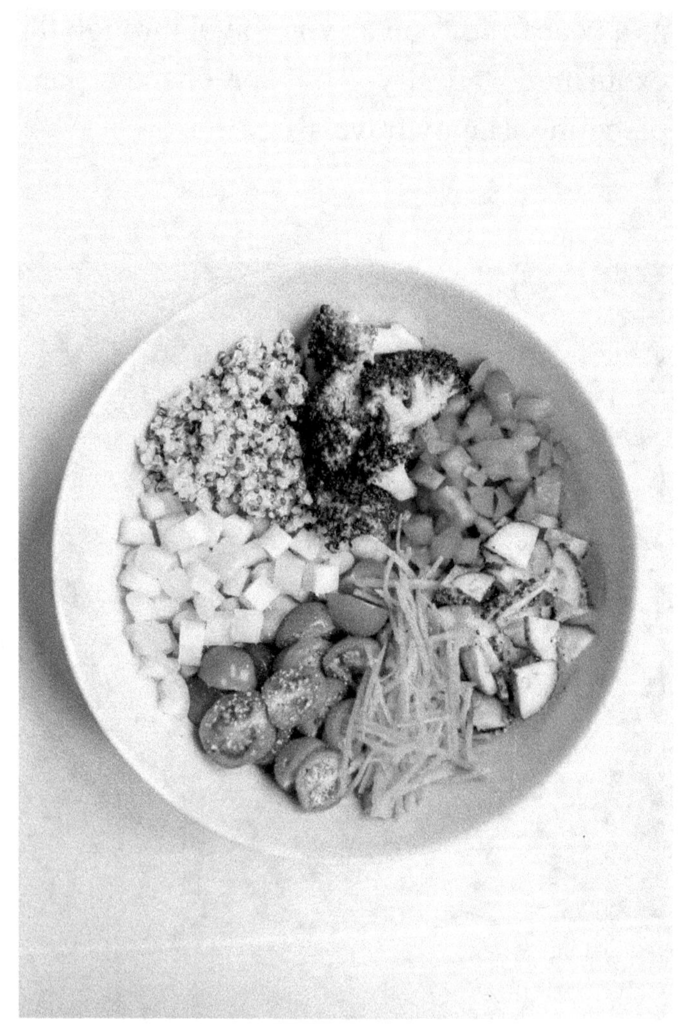

Chapter One

Understanding Gestational Diabetes

The groundwork for our investigation of gestational diabetes, a distinct kind of diabetes that develops during pregnancy, is laid out in Chapter 1. We examine gestational diabetes' definition, prevalence, risk factors, and possible effects on both the mother and the fetus. Understanding this disease is essential because it equips expectant mothers with the knowledge and instruments they need to appropriately manage their health during this life-changing period.

1.1 Gestational Diabetes Defined

We describe gestational diabetes and outline how it differs from other kinds of diabetes in this section. When the body is unable to create enough insulin to control blood sugar levels during pregnancy, gestational diabetes develops. Around 2-10% of pregnancies worldwide are affected by it, which often manifests during the second or third trimester.

1.2 Frequency and Risk Elements

We examine the prevalence of gestational diabetes while taking into account that it occurs at diverse rates in various demographics and geographical areas. We go over the risk factors that can make gestational diabetes more likely to occur, including the mother's age, family history of diabetes, obesity, and prior gestational diabetes.

1.3 The Value of Pregnancy Diabetes Management

The importance of treating gestational diabetes is emphasized in this section to encourage a healthy pregnancy for both the mother and the unborn child. Neglecting to properly treat gestational diabetes can result in issues including high birth weight, neonatal hypoglycemia, and a higher chance of both the mother and the child later in life acquiring type 2 diabetes. To reduce these hazards, we emphasize the value of early discovery, ongoing observation, and effective management.

1.4 Screening and Diagnosis

We review the many screening techniques for gestational diabetes, such as the oral glucose tolerance test (OGTT) and the glucose challenge test (GCT), as we explore the diagnosis procedure. We offer details on how medical professionals interpret the findings and the actions followed following a diagnosis to properly manage the disease.

1.5 Nutritional Management of Gestational Diabetes

We promote the notion of utilizing diet as the major strategy to control blood sugar levels since nutrition is vital in treating gestational diabetes. We explore the role of carbs, proteins, and fats in the diet and how they affect blood sugar levels while emphasizing the need for balanced meals. A healthy pregnancy and blood sugar levels can both be supported by a well-managed diet.

1.6 Cooperative Support and Care

We emphasize the necessity of collaborative care in controlling gestational diabetes while highlighting the value of collaboration. We urge women who are expecting to consult closely with their medical professionals, such as obstetricians, endocrinologists, and registered dietitians, to develop individualized care plans that are catered to their particular needs. We also go over the importance of getting help from loved ones, friends, and support groups to maintain mental health when traveling.

A call to action for pregnant people to actively manage gestational diabetes by embracing nutrition as a potent weapon in their pregnancy journey is presented at the end of Chapter 1. Understanding the effects of gestational diabetes gives women the power to take control of their health, guaranteeing a better and easier pregnancy experience for both them and their priceless unborn children. The information learned in this chapter acts as a guide for the chapters to follow, where we'll get into the details of dietary remedies for conditions like gestational diabetes, nausea, and edema to promote a positive and loving pregnant experience.

Swelling22

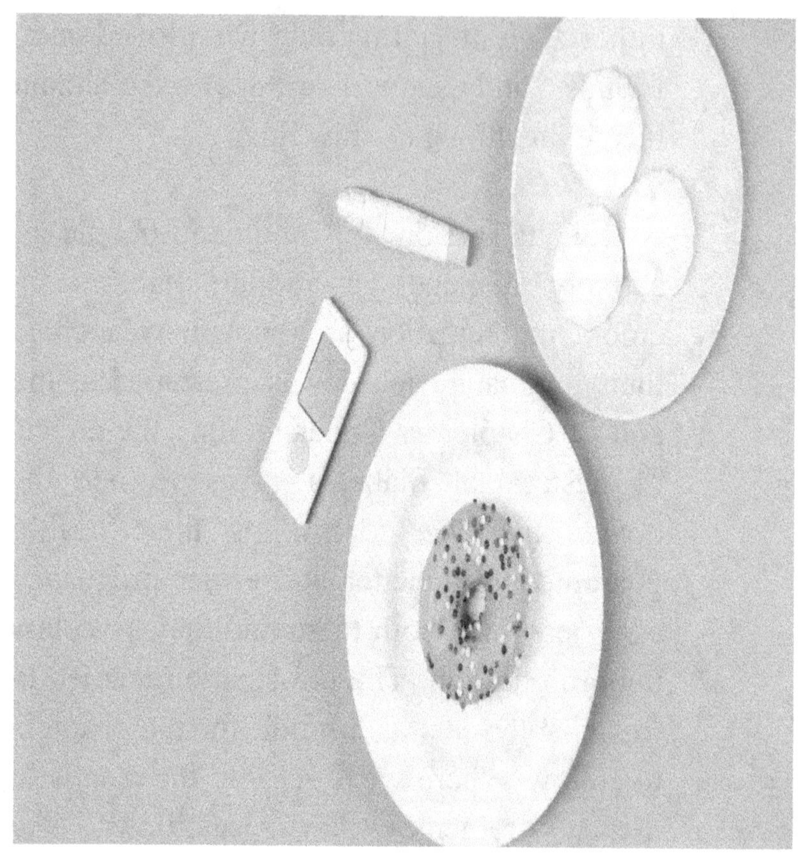

Chapter Two

Navigating Gestational Diabetes: Basic Nutrition Information

The fundamentals of dietary management for gestational diabetes are covered in Chapter 2. We set out on a voyage across the world of carbs, proteins, and fats to comprehend their effects on the health of pregnant women generally and blood sugar levels in particular. Understanding these nutritional fundamentals helps expectant mothers make wise dietary decisions that support a healthy pregnancy and stable blood sugar levels.

2.1   Dietary Management of Gestational Diabetes

In this part, we examine how important nutrition is to controlling gestational diabetes. To regulate blood sugar levels and reduce pregnancy problems, a proper diet is essential. We stress the importance of using food as medicine and draw attention to the fact that even little dietary changes can have a big influence on general health.

2.2   Recognizing Blood Glucose Levels and Their Importance

Understanding blood sugar levels and their effects is crucial for managing gestational diabetes. We go through the usual range of blood glucose levels during pregnancy, how changes might happen, and how crucial it is to keep levels steady for both the mother and the unborn child.

2.3 The Energy Source Is Carbohydrates:

Carbohydrates are essential for controlling blood sugar levels. We examine several carbohydrate kinds, including basic and complex carbs, and how they affect blood sugar levels. To maintain stable blood sugar levels, readers learn how to recognize healthy carbohydrate sources and control portion sizes.

2.4 Proteins: Health's Building Blocks

The discussion of proteins and their importance during pregnancy is covered in the next chapter. We talk about how proteins support the baby's healthy growth and development while stabilizing blood sugar levels. Pregnant women can maximize their nutrient intake by using lean protein sources in their diet.

2.5 Fats: Crucial for Maintaining Hormonal Balance

The significance of fats in promoting hormonal balance and general health during pregnancy is the main topic of this section. We make a distinction between good and bad fats and offer advice to readers on how to include healthy fats in their diets. In addition, we describe how necessary fatty acids help a baby's developing brain.

2.6 Maintaining a Balance of Carbohydrates, Proteins, and Fats

In this section, we integrate our understanding of carbs, proteins, and fats to show how these three macronutrients work together to maintain blood sugar levels. The proper ratio of these macronutrients will be included in balanced meals that readers learn how to make, enabling better blood glucose regulation.

2.7 Mindful Eating for Pregnancy-Related Diabetes

A key component of treating gestational diabetes is attentive eating. By introducing the idea of mindful eating, we hope to inspire readers to pay attention and be present when they eat. Recognizing hunger cues, preventing overeating, and creating a healthy connection with food are all made possible by mindful eating.

2.8 Nutritional Management of Gestational Diabetes: Useful Advice

We provide helpful advice for treating gestational diabetes through diet in the chapter's conclusion. These recommendations could include techniques for meal preparation, adding frequent snacks, and keeping a food journal to track dietary decisions and blood sugar reactions. We also urge women who are expecting to develop individualized dietary regimens in collaboration with certified dietitians and medical professionals.

Understanding the fundamentals of nutrition is a great tool for treating gestational diabetes and supporting a healthy pregnancy, as Chapter 2 concludes. Understanding the functions of carbs, proteins, and fats enables pregnant people to make educated meal decisions that support stable blood sugar levels, improve general well-being, and nurture the priceless life inside. As we go on to the next chapters, readers will discover thorough advice and doable solutions to deal with the unique difficulties of pregnancy swelling and nausea, promoting a peaceful and satisfying pregnant experience.

Chapter Three

Making a Meal Plan for Gestational Diabetes

In Chapter 3, we set out on a personal nutrition journey and create a specialized food plan to help us confidently navigate the seas of gestational diabetes. We recognize that each pregnant experience and the dietary path that goes along with it are distinct as we map this road. We will assist women who are pregnant in creating a food plan that maintains stable blood sugar levels, provides necessary nutrients, and promotes a healthy and joyful pregnancy using the compass of knowledge and the spirit of creativity.

3.1 Determining Each Person's Nutritional Needs

The importance of determining each person's unique dietary needs is emphasized at the beginning of the chapter. We acknowledge that each pregnant person has unique nutritional needs depending on things like age, weight, degree of exercise, and general health. We go through the significance of working together with registered dietitians and medical professionals to develop a tailored meal plan that caters to these special requirements.

3.2 Construction of a Balanced Plate

With an emphasis on the ratios of carbs, proteins, and fats, we explore the art of creating a balanced meal. To encourage stable blood sugar levels, we offer recommendations for portion control and the distribution of nutrients throughout the day. The book's readers will discover how to prepare meals that are filling, healthy, and supportive of their wellness objectives.

3.3 Choosing Foods with a Low Glycemic Index

We present the idea of the glycemic index (GI) to successfully control gestational diabetes. We advise readers to choose low-GI meals since they digest more slowly and cause blood sugar levels to rise gradually. We look at several low-GI food selections and how they fit into the meal plan.

3.4 Highlighting Foods High in Fiber

An important component of the meal plan is including foods that are high in fiber. We go through how dietary fiber helps digestion, maintains steady blood sugar levels, and prevents constipation. We discuss several foods high in fiber and inventive methods to include them in everyday meals.

3.5 Wise Snacking Techniques

Snacking is essential for regulating nutritional intake and treating gestational diabetes. We provide sage snacking advice, such as the recommendation of snacks that are well-balanced and contain carbs, protein, and good fats. These snacks help keep blood sugar stable in between meals while also satisfying hunger.

3.6 Maintaining Hydration and Blood Sugar

The chapter examines how hydration affects controlling blood sugar. For women who are gestational diabetic and pregnant, drinking the right amount of fluids is essential. We go through the importance of water, herbal teas, and other hydrating drinks while also offering advice on how to stay properly hydrated all day long.

3.7 Sample Menus & Meal Plan Examples

We provide sample menus and meal plan samples to illustrate the meal planning procedure. These inventive and varied meal suggestions, which cover a range of cultures and flavors, will inspire readers. These illustrations show the adaptability and depth of a thoughtfully created gestational diabetic meal plan.

3.8 The Influence of Meal Planning

An important skill in treating gestational diabetes is meal preparation. We provide advice and methods for efficient meal preparation, such as batch cooking, meal planning for hectic days, and inventive leftover utilization. Food preparation makes it easier to stick to a food plan and promotes consistency.

The encouraging message that finishes Chapter 3 is that creating a gestational diabetes meal plan is an art that reflects unique requirements, preferences, and objectives. Pregnant women may go on a culinary adventure that not only controls gestational diabetes but also feeds the body and spirit during the pregnancy journey by combining knowledge, creativity, and assistance from healthcare professionals. To ensure a thorough and enriching approach to fostering a healthy and enjoyable pregnancy, we will dive into managing nausea and swelling during pregnancy as we move through the next chapters.

Chapter Four

Managing Nausea During Pregnancy

The turbulent waters of pregnancy sickness, a major worry for many pregnant women, are explored in Chapter 4. We recognize that navigating through these waves can be difficult, but have no fear—we are armed with a wealth of nutritional ideas and doable advice to help you feel better and make your pregnant journey more bearable. We traverse this chapter to help pregnant people get rid of their motion sicknesses and enjoy the benefits of being pregnant.

4.1 Recognizing Nausea During Pregnancy

The first section of the chapter explains morning sickness, another name for pregnant nausea. We look at its prevalence, typical causes, and the range of severity that various people experience. Understanding the nature of pregnant sickness helps readers understand why it happens and how it could affect their general well-being.

4.2   Nutritional   Techniques   to Reduce Nausea

We discover a wealth of dietary tactics that may be used to traverse the nausea seas of pregnancy. We talk about the advantages of eating small, frequent meals and including ginger in your diet since it has anti-nausea effects. We also look at additional stomach-soothing and discomfort-reducing anti-nausea meals and drinks.

4.3 Hydration Is Important

Keeping hydrated becomes essential while experiencing waves of nausea. We stress the importance of being properly hydrated throughout pregnancy since it reduces nausea and preserves general well-being. We provide advice on how to consume hydrating liquids all day long and examine the advantages of herbal teas and other non-caffeinated beverages.

4.4 Nutrient-Dense Foods for Relief from Nausea

We provide nutrient-rich foods that help reduce pregnancy sickness while navigating the dietary seas. We examine how magnesium, vitamin B6, and other crucial minerals support healthy digestion and lessen motion sickness. Pregnant women might comfort themselves in feeding their bodies when feeling ill by including these items in their diet.

4.5 Reduce Triggers

This section covers techniques for locating and reducing factors that aggravate nausea. We investigate the effects of strong scents, specific meals, and ambient elements on nausea during pregnancy. With this knowledge, readers may modify their environment and food preferences to make it more nausea-friendly.

4.6 Managing Nausea: Emotional Assistance

We understand the emotional component of dealing with morning sickness when pregnant in addition to nutrition solutions. We talk about how vital emotional support from spouses, relatives, and friends is. To manage stress and maintain emotional health, we also look at mindfulness practices, relaxation exercises, and other coping tactics.

4.7 Useful Advice for Scheduling Meals While Nauseous

We provide useful advice and suggestions to assist pregnant women who are experiencing nausea through meal planning. We advise them to be flexible with mealtimes, concentrate on preparing straightforward, readily digested meals, and eat comforting and reviving foods.

4.8 Seeking Expert Assistance

The need of getting expert assistance if nausea becomes severe or chronic is emphasized as the chapter comes to a close. We urge women who are expecting to speak with their doctors to rule out any underlying conditions and look at other possible courses of therapy.

The conclusion of Chapter 4 gives the comfort that treating morning sickness during pregnancy is possible with the proper dietary techniques and mental support. As we continue on this journey, we honor pregnant women's fortitude, bravery, and capacity to gracefully and resolutely ride the waves of sickness. We set sail to investigate the area of controlling edema during pregnancy with the compass of dietary solutions and support, enhancing our voyage with knowledge and empowerment.

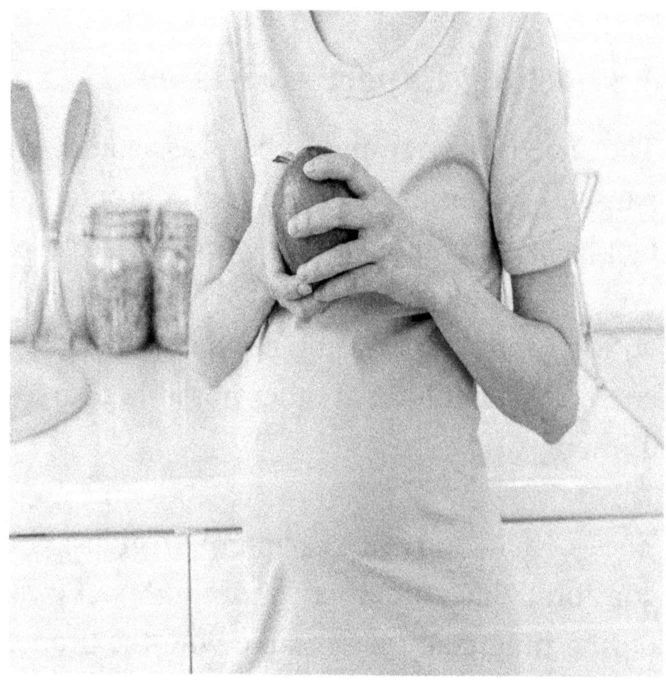

Chapter Five

Nutritional Treatments for Swelling and Fluid Retention

We set sail on a journey in Chapter 5 to tackle the typical worry of edema and fluid retention during pregnancy. We are aware that swelling is sometimes a normal aspect of pregnancy as we navigate these waters, but severe or unexpected swelling may call for medical care. We provide expectant women with a wealth of dietary strategies and self-care techniques to properly manage swelling and foster general well-being during their pregnancy.

5.1 Pregnancy Edema: What to Know

The discussion of edema, the medical term for swelling brought on by fluid retention, opens the chapter. We talk about the physiological alterations, such as increased blood volume and hormonal changes, that result in edema during pregnancy. Knowing the characteristics of edema can help you determine when it is normal and when it needs further attention.

5.2 Knowing When to Pay Attention to Swelling

To help patients navigate the waters of edema, we've highlighted certain signs and symptoms that may indicate when swelling calls for medical treatment. The distinction between normal and severe swelling is discussed, and it is emphasized that if swelling is accompanied by other symptoms or unexpected changes, it is crucial to seek expert advice.

5.3 Dietary Supplements and Foods to Reduce Swelling

By using nutrition as our compass, we may navigate through edema by examining foods and nutrients that can assist to lessen swelling. We emphasize the importance of foods high in potassium for maintaining healthy fluid balance and promoting renal function. We also offer foods that have anti-inflammatory qualities that might help to reduce edema.

5.4 Limiting Sodium Consumption

This section examines methods for controlling sodium consumption during pregnancy and discusses the function of sodium in fluid retention. Pregnant women can maintain a healthy balance and reduce edema by making thoughtful meal choices and being aware of hidden sources of salt.

5.5 Recommendations for Hydration and Fluid Intake

To manage edema, proper hydration is essential. We talk about the significance of maintaining the fluid balance between intake and outflow as well as remaining hydrated. We also look at the advantages of hydrating meals and drinks, which can improve general health and lessen edema.

5.6 Exercises Pregnancy-Friendly for Swelling

We consider dietary alternatives while also acknowledging the value of exercise in treating edema. We go through easy activities that are safe for pregnant women and increase circulation while decreasing fluid retention. Pregnant women should supplement dietary efforts to control edema by including safe physical exercise in their regimen.

5.7 Raising and Reposing

In addition to diet and exercise, we recognize the value of elevating and sleeping as self-care activities to reduce edema. We look at methods for reducing edema and promoting comfort while resting frequently and elevating the feet.

5.8 Collaborative Care for the Management of Swelling

A reminder of the need for coordinated care in controlling edema is provided in the chapter's conclusion. We urge expectant mothers to collaborate closely with medical professionals, such as obstetricians, midwives, and qualified dietitians, to develop a comprehensive strategy for controlling swelling and enhancing general well-being.

The lesson of Chapter 5 is that minimizing edema during pregnancy requires self-care and empowerment. Pregnant women may sail the waves of edema with confidence and grace by using the compass of dietary strategies and self-care techniques. As our trip continues, we will delve further into the world of pregnant superfoods, enhancing it with the strength of sustenance and fortitude.

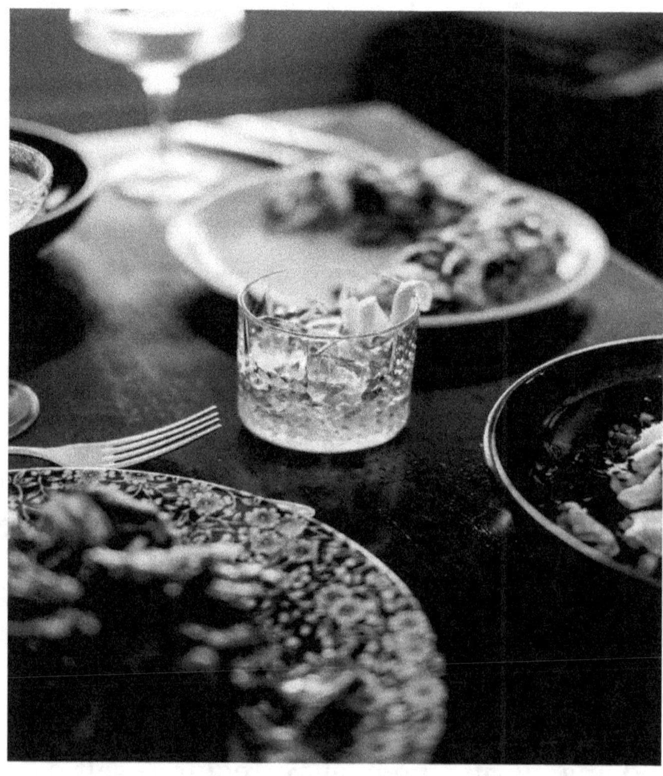

Chapter Six

Pregnancy Superfoods: A Nutrient Powerhouse

We set off on a voyage into the opulent world of pregnancy superfoods in Chapter 6, a treasure trove of nutrient-rich treats that sustain both the expecting woman and the developing baby. We realize that these superfoods' extraordinary nutritional profile, which provides a symphony of vitamins, minerals, antioxidants, and other necessary elements, is what gives them their magic. To ensure a journey of optimal nourishment and well-being, we will study a variety of pregnant superfoods, their health advantages, and innovative methods to include them in the diet as we proceed through this chapter.

6.1 The Pregnancy Superfoods' Power

The notion of pregnancy superfoods and their importance in boosting mother and fetal health are introduced at the beginning of the chapter. We examine the nutritional qualities that distinguish these foods, such as their high concentrations of folate, iron, calcium, omega-3 fatty acids, and other elements vital for a healthy pregnancy.

Leafy greens are one of nature's nutrient-dense gems.
We delve into the realm of leafy greens in this part, including spinach, kale, and Swiss chard. We emphasize the amount of antioxidants, vitamins, and minerals they contain, such as folate, vitamin K, iron, and vitamin C. The advantages of leafy greens in promoting healthy prenatal development and lowering the likelihood of specific birth abnormalities will be revealed to readers.

6.3   Berries: Packed   with Antioxidants

As we navigate the world of prenatal superfoods, we come across the colorful world of berries, which are some of nature's most potent sources of antioxidants. We talk about the berries' high vitamin C content, fiber content, and other phytonutrients, which enhance immune health and general well-being.

6.4 Nuts and seeds are a natural source of protein and good fats.

In this part, we examine the protein-, fat-, and nutrient-rich gem that is nuts and seeds. We go through the advantages of including foods like flaxseeds, chia seeds, almonds, and walnuts in the diet since they boost brain growth and are a good source of plant-based omega-3 fatty acids.

6.5 Omega-3-Rich Delicacies, such as Fatty Fish

We come across fatty fish like salmon, mackerel, and trout, which are rife with omega-3 fatty acids while navigating the oceans of pregnant superfoods. In addition to discussing the possible advantages of lowering the risk of preterm delivery, we also explore the significance of omega-3s in embryonic brain and eye development.

6.6 Legumes: Powerhouses of Protein and Fiber

We discover the nutritious gems of legumes, such as lentils, chickpeas, and black beans, as we continue our journey. We look at how the abundance of plant-based protein, fiber, iron, and folate makes them an important addition to the diet during pregnancy.

6.7 Calcium from Dairy Promotes Strong Bones

We set sail across the world of dairy in this part as a source of calcium for healthy bones and teeth. We talk about the significance of calcium during pregnancy for the skeletal development of both the mother and the fetus.

6.8 Pregnancy Superfood Recipes and Meal Ideas

We provide a variety of delectable dishes and meal suggestions to bring the magic of pregnant superfoods to life. Dishes that use leafy greens, berries, nuts, seeds, and fatty fish will inspire readers and make it simple to enjoy the benefits of these nutritional powerhouses.

6.9 Choosing Variety for Best Nutrition

The chapter ends by reminding readers how important it is to eat a varied diet to get the advantages of several pregnancy superfoods. We advise women who are expecting to combine several superfoods to create a symphony of tastes and nutrition that will benefit both their health and the growth of their unborn child.

Lists of Healthful Superfoods for Pregnancy and Their Categories

1. Leafy Greens: Crucial nutrients for fetal growth and general health include folate, iron, calcium, and vitamins A, C, and K, which are abundant in spinach, kale, Swiss chard, and collard greens.

2. Berries: Blueberries, strawberries, raspberries, and blackberries are loaded with antioxidants, vitamin C, and fiber, all of which enhance immune function and supply essential nutrients.

3. Almonds, walnuts, chia seeds, and flaxseeds are wonderful sources of protein, good fats, and necessary elements, such as omega-3 fatty acids that boost brain development.

4. Fatty Fish: Omega-3 fatty acids, which are critical for the development of the embryonic brain and eyes, are abundant in salmon, mackerel, and trout.

5. Legumes: Peas, black beans, lentils, and chickpeas are high in iron, folate, fiber, and plant-based protein, supporting the health of both the mother and the fetus.

6. Dairy: Milk, yogurt, and cheese are great sources of calcium, which is necessary for both the mother and the fetus to develop strong bones and teeth.

7. Avocado: Rich in critical minerals like potassium and folate as well as fiber and good fats, avocados are a pregnant woman's best friend.

8. Sweet potatoes: are an excellent source of beta-carotene, a substance that the body converts to vitamin A and is crucial for the growth and development of the fetus.

9. Eggs: Choline, which is necessary for healthy brain development and overall well-being, is also found in eggs, making them a complete protein source.

10. Quinoa: this is an excellent addition to the diet during pregnancy since it is a nutrient-dense grain that is high in protein, fiber, and several vitamins and minerals.

11. Greek yogurt: Greek yogurt is a source of vital nutrients and is high in protein, calcium, and probiotics, all of which help digestive health.

12. Oranges: Citrus fruits, such as oranges, are rich in vitamin C, which boosts the immune system and helps the body absorb iron.

13. Broccoli: Packed in calcium, iron, vitamins C, K, and folate, broccoli is a nutritious powerhouse.

14. Legumes: Legumes are a great source of plant-based protein, iron, and fiber and they also contribute to a diet that is well-balanced during pregnancy.

15. Chia Seeds: Chia seeds are a fantastic source of calcium, fiber, and omega-3 fatty acids, giving pregnant women a nutritional boost.

The celebration of pregnancy superfoods, nature's nutritious powerhouses that provide pregnant women with the best nutrition and vigor, marks the conclusion of Chapter 6. Pregnant women may enhance their prenatal journey with a cornucopia of vitamins, minerals, and antioxidants that support maternal and fetal health by including these jewels into their diet. As we go on, we'll investigate how exercise might help you deal with pregnancy-related worries and build resilience as you embark on the life-changing experience of becoming a mother.

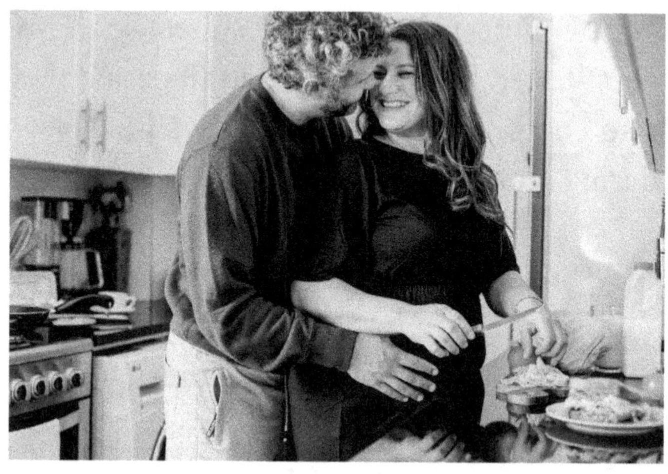

Chapter Seven

Exercise's Function in Managing Pregnancy Concerns

In Chapter 7, expectant women are encouraged to embrace exercise's transforming potential as a crucial management strategy for pregnancy-related anxieties. We set out on a trip that emphasizes the many advantages of pregnancy-friendly physical activity, learning how it may help with gestational diabetes management, relieve nausea, lessen swelling, and promote general well-being. As we progress through this chapter, we learn how diet and exercise work together to allow pregnant people to set out on a balanced and active journey toward a healthier and more satisfying pregnancy experience.

7.1 Recognizing Exercise Safe for Pregnancy

Beginning with a discussion on pregnancy-friendly exercise, the chapter acknowledges the need for a thoughtful and specialized approach to physical activity during pregnancy. We examine the recommendations for safe and suitable exercise throughout various phases of pregnancy, urging readers to speak with medical professionals to find workouts fit for their particular requirements and medical background.

7.2 Exercise Management for Gestational Diabetes

We discuss how exercise can help manage gestational diabetes in this section. In this article, we'll look at how exercise can enhance insulin sensitivity, control blood sugar levels, and aid in overall glucose management. The activities the readers learn can be incorporated into their regular routines to support a healthy and balanced pregnancy.

7.3 Relieving Nausea by Moving Around

We investigate how exercise might reduce pregnant sickness as we navigate the world of fitness. We go through easy workouts that improve circulation, soothe gastrointestinal pain, and lessen the severity of morning sickness. We compassionately urge women who are pregnant to listen to their bodies and select workouts that feel relaxing and comfortable.

7.4 Lessening Fluid Retention and Swelling with Movement

We study how physical activity might help to assist in the decrease of edema and fluid retention during pregnancy by navigating the waters of exercise. We go through activities that assist in the treatment of edema by promoting circulation and lymphatic drainage. We advise pregnant women to put their comfort and safety first, emphasizing low-impact activities.

7.5 Combining relaxation with mindfulness

We examine the benefits of mindfulness and relaxation techniques when exercising in addition to the physical side. To improve readers' experiences exercising, we lead them through mindful movement routines that incorporate deep breathing, visualization, and relaxation techniques.

7.6 Prenatal Pilates and Prenatal Yoga

We set sail through the worlds of prenatal Pilates and yoga in this part. We examine the advantages of these targeted, mild activities that promote emotional stability, strength, and flexibility during pregnancy. The mind-body connection that is cultivated by these activities will be an encouragement to expectant mothers.

7.7 Collaborating with Healthcare Professionals

The chapter emphasizes the value of working together with healthcare professionals to create an activity plan that complies with specific health requirements and pregnancy-related worries. We go through the value of being honest with medical experts and the advantages of getting advice on the activities that are most appropriate for each person's stage of pregnancy.

7.8 Maintaining Hydration and Nutrition

We continue to highlight how important it is to be hydrated and fed when exercising. To sustain energy levels and promote overall well-being, it's important to drink the right amount of water and eat mindfully before and after physical exercise.

The appreciation of the transformational impact of exercise during pregnancy marks the end of Chapter 7. Pregnant people can successfully traverse the rough waters of gestational diabetes, nausea, and edema by adopting pregnancy-friendly physical exercise. We set sail on the maternal journey to study the skill of managing food aversions and cravings using the combination of nutrition and exercise as our compass.

Chapter Eight

Managing Food Cravings and Aversions During Pregnancy

The interesting and frequently unpredictable world of pregnancy-related food desires and aversions is explored in Chapter 8. We are aware that this journey can be difficult for some pregnant women as they deal with unanticipated appetites and aversions to once-favorite foods. In this chapter, we examine the science underlying these modifications and provide compassionate ways to manage cravings and food aversions while still eating a nutritious and well-balanced diet during pregnancy.

8.1 Recognizing Food Cravings and Aversions

The first section of the chapter explores the hormonal and physiological changes that cause food cravings and aversions during pregnancy. We go into how these preferences are shaped by pregnant hormones and the senses to assist readers realize that these sensations are a normal part of the journey.

8.2 Managing Food Aversions

We provide compassionate advice to deal with these abrupt dislikes of food while navigating the waters of food aversions. Pregnant women are urged to accept flexibility in their eating plans and look into substitute foods that offer comparable nutrition. Despite aversions, people can maintain a balanced and diverse diet by remaining open to exploring new flavors and sensations.

8.3 Mindfully navigating cravings

In this part, we examine the idea of mindful eating and how it may be used to manage cravings for certain foods while pregnant. We advise women who are expecting to pay attention to their bodies and comprehend the meanings behind their wants. They may indulge in their favorite foods while putting their overall nutrition first if they give in to their impulses in moderation and balance.

8.4 Keeping Nutritional Needs in Check

We emphasize the significance of balancing nutritional demands as we navigate the world of food aversions and urges. We talk about the importance of essential nutrients including folate, iron, calcium, and omega-3 fatty acids during pregnancy. Even in the face of shifting taste preferences, pregnant women will find inspiration in innovative methods to include nutrient-rich foods in their diet.

8.5 Adopting Snacking and Hydration

During this journey, it is even more important to stay hydrated and eat regularly. We go through the advantages of hydrating drinks like water and herbal teas as a supplement to the pregnant woman's diet. Additionally, we provide suggestions for nutrient-dense snacks that fulfill appetites throughout pregnancy.

8.6 Locating Understanding and Support

We underscore the value of getting help and understanding throughout this section. People's responses to a pregnant person's appetites and aversions might vary widely. To foster a welcoming environment that respects each person's individual experiences, we promote open conversation with partners, family, and healthcare professionals.

8.7 Preparing Food and Meals for Cravings and Aversions:

We provide cooking and meal preparation advice that takes shifting taste preferences into account to bring the journey of food aversions and desires to life. We look at the advantages of including family members and partners in meal preparation to encourage a cooperative and supportive approach to nourishing the expecting woman.

8.8 Getting Expert Advice

The chapter ends by stressing the value of getting expert guidance if food aversions or cravings become out of control or have an impact on general nutrition. We advise women who are expecting to speak with licensed dietitians or other medical professionals to make sure they are getting enough nutrition and managing their diets properly.

The celebration of the complex and dynamic journey of food aversions and desires throughout pregnancy marks the conclusion of Chapter 8. Pregnant women may successfully navigate these waters by embracing adaptability, mindfulness, and support. The importance of being properly hydrated throughout pregnancy will be discussed as we go forth, reviving our spirits with water's lifeblood and nurturing our bodies on this transforming parenthood journey.

Chapter Nine

The Lifeline of Pregnancy: The Importance of Proper Hydration

Proper hydration, a crucial component that maintains and feeds the expecting mother and her developing baby, is celebrated in Chapter 9 as the lifeline of pregnancy. As we set out on this journey, we are aware of the crucial part that water plays in maintaining pregnant health, encouraging healthy body processes, and boosting overall well-being. In this chapter, we examine the importance of staying hydrated throughout pregnancy, look at the advantages of water, herbal teas, and hydrating meals, and provide doable tips for doing so.

9.1 The Benefits of Staying Hydrated During Pregnancy

An examination of the significance of water during pregnancy opens the chapter. We go through the physiological alterations that take place during pregnancy, such as the rise in blood volume and amniotic fluid, which call for a greater intake of fluids. Readers will see water as a priceless resource on their pregnant journey after learning how hydration supports overall wellness.

9.2 Water's Health Benefits for Mother and Baby

We explore the many advantages of water for both the expecting mother and the unborn child as we navigate the waters of hydration. We go through how enough hydration promotes healthy digestion, lowers the risk of uTIs, assists in maintaining body warmth, and supports amniotic fluid levels, which are crucial for fetal development.

9.3 Natural Nutritious Drinks: Herbal Teas and Infusions

We examine herbal teas and infusions in this area as a hydrating and reviving choice for pregnant women. We emphasize the range of herbal teas on the market, each of which has special health advantages. These healthy drinks can be incorporated into a pregnant person's everyday routine as inspiration.

9.4 Foods that Hydrate for Best Nutrition

We learn about the variety of hydrating meals that may be consumed in addition to fluid consumption as we navigate the world of hydration. We examine fruits and vegetables that are high in water content since they not only quench thirst but also offer vital vitamins, minerals, and antioxidants. These savory and hydrating meals will be a treat for pregnant women to nurture their bodies with.

9.5 Meeting Hydration Needs During Pregnancy

We offer suggestions in this area for ensuring that hydration requirements are met at various stages of pregnancy. We go through how crucial it is to modify fluid intake according to one's activity level, the weather, and personal requirements. Pregnant women should be well-hydrated on their parenthood journey by paying attention to their thirst cues.

9.6 Realistic Techniques for Remaining Hydrated

We provide helpful advice and suggestions for staying hydrated during pregnancy to assist in navigating the waters of optimal hydration. We go through the importance of keeping a water bottle with you, setting reminders for regular hydration, and including hydrating foods and drinks in meals and snacks.

9.7 Keeping Hydrated While Traveling

As we go on, we investigate how to remain hydrated while on the road. We go through methods for keeping fluid intake consistent amid hectic schedules and provide advice on how to pick hydrated foods whether traveling or dining out.

9.8 Obtaining Expert Advice

The chapter's conclusion emphasizes the significance of seeing a specialist for advice on hydration requirements if pregnant women have certain medical issues or worries. We support open dialogue with medical professionals and certified dietitians to customize fluid intake to specific health needs.

A celebration of good hydration, a priceless resource that feeds and supports the pregnant woman and her unborn child, marks the conclusion of Chapter 9. It is the lifeline of pregnancy. Pregnant women may embark on this life-changing journey with vigor and well-being if they understand the importance of water and hydrating meals. As we move further on our journey, we will investigate the practice of self-care throughout pregnancy, nourishing the body as well as the soul as we approach the closing chapters of this fruitful and transformational journey known as motherhood.

Chapter Ten

The Art of Self-Care During Pregnancy: Nurturing Body and Soul.

Pregnant women are invited to go on a journey of nourishing their bodies and souls in Chapter 10, which honors the art of self-care throughout pregnancy. We are aware that being pregnant is a life-changing experience that calls for compassion, mindfulness, and self-awareness. This chapter examines the necessity of self-care throughout pregnancy and provides doable methods for putting one's physical, emotional, and mental well-being first. Pregnant women who set out on this journey of self-love and care can discover comfort, resiliency, and fulfillment as they travel the path to motherhood.

10.1 Self-Care is Important During Pregnancy

An examination of the value of self-care during pregnancy opens the chapter. We talk about how practicing self-care fosters one's physical, and emotional, and facilitates a smooth and satisfying pregnant experience. Readers will appreciate the importance of self-care once they comprehend how crucial it is to enjoy the life-changing experience of pregnancy.

10.2 Giving rest and sleep a priority:

We emphasize the value of relaxation and sleep throughout pregnancy as we navigate the waters of self-care. We go over the physiological changes that might impact sleep habits and provide tips for encouraging restful sleep. Pregnant women can promote a feeling of renewal and vigor by prioritizing rest and fostering a peaceful sleep environment.

10.3 Gentle movement and exercise:

This section examines the benefits of light exercise and movement for prenatal self-care. We talk about pregnancy-friendly activities that promote both physical and mental wellness, such as yoga, swimming, and walking. By embracing the joy of exercise, pregnant women can improve their journey by feeling more alive and connected to their bodies.

10.4 Relaxation and mindfulness exercises:

We explore soul-nourishing mindfulness and relaxation techniques as we navigate the self-care landscape. We look at deep breathing, visualization, and meditation techniques to provide expectant women skills to calm down, create emotional balance, and reduce stress.

10.5 Explicit Emotional Expression and Support-Seeking:

In this part, we stress the importance of talking about your feelings and getting assistance when you're pregnant. We urge women who are pregnant, to be honest about their experiences and feelings with their partners, families, and friends. They can successfully negotiate the emotional waters of pregnancy by developing a support system and, if necessary, obtaining expert assistance.

10.6 Establishing a Protective and Supportive Environment:

We talk about the need of providing a secure and supportive atmosphere throughout pregnancy as we navigate the waters of self-care. We look at the advantages of being surrounded by supportive people, pursuing artistic endeavors, and bringing joy and comfort into everyday life.

10.7 Feeding Your Body Nutrient-Rich Foods:

We emphasize the significance of providing the body with nutrient-rich meals as we go forward on our journey. We celebrate the strength of hydrating foods and superfoods during pregnancy that provides the body with crucial nutrients and promotes overall health and energy.

10.8 Learning to Have Self-Compassion

The celebration of self-compassion as a crucial component of self-care marks the chapter's conclusion. We urge women who are pregnant to practice self-compassion and let go of self-criticism. They may enter the changing journey of motherhood with grace and resiliency by cultivating a kind and loving relationship with themselves.

The celebration of the art of self-care throughout pregnancy, a journey of nurturing the body and spirit with compassion, awareness, and alertness, marks the conclusion of Chapter 10. Pregnant women can successfully navigate the waters of pregnancy by emphasizing relaxation, taking part in mild exercise, and fostering emotional well-being. As we go on our trip, we'll examine the art of labor preparation and equip expectant women with information and support as they set out on the last leg of this life-changing motherhood journey.

Chapter Eleven

Empowering Birth Plans and Supportive Strategies for Preparing for Childbirth

In Chapter 11, the transforming process of getting ready for labor is explored, arming pregnant moms with information, assurance, and supporting techniques. We recognize that giving birth is a special and personalized event and that each person's journey deserves to be honored and respected. This chapter discusses the significance of birth planning, birthing education, emotional support, and coping mechanisms for navigating labor and accepting this life-changing experience.

11.1 Recognizing the Childbirth Experience

The chapter opens with an examination of the delivery process, paying tribute to the tenacity and fortitude of pregnant women as they approach this important milestone. Our discussion of the many stages of labor, such as early labor, active labor, and the pushing stage, equips readers to accept delivery naturally with bravery and amazement.

11.2 The Birth Plans' Empowerment

In this part, we emphasize the value of birth plans, which provide expectant women the freedom to voice their choices and aspirations for their labor and delivery experiences. We go through the elements of a birth plan, such as pain relief alternatives, laboring positions, and birthing location preferences. Expectant moms can approach labor with confidence and a sense of control over their experience by embracing the power of choice.

11.3 Preparation and education for childbirth

We examine the usefulness of birthing education programs while navigating the waters of prenatal care. We go through the advantages of becoming familiar with labor physiology, pain relief methods, breathing exercises, and coping mechanisms. Expectant moms can approach labor with a sense of readiness and understanding by arming themselves with information.

11.4 Labor-Related Coping Strategies

In this part, we examine coping mechanisms for reducing pain and suffering during childbirth. We look at breathing exercises, massages, visualization methods, and relaxation techniques to provide expecting moms and their birth partners with a toolbox of skills to employ throughout labor.

11.5 Emotional assistance throughout labor

We become more and more aware of the need for emotional support throughout labor as we navigate the waters of childbirth. We talk about the support, solace, and advocacy that birth partners, doulas, and medical professionals may offer. An encouraging delivery team that respects the preferences and requirements of the expectant woman will provide them comfort.

11.6 Taking the Unexpected in stride

In this part, we examine the value of flexibility and adaptation while embracing the unpredictable nature of labor. We consider the idea of submitting to the birthing process while acknowledging that it could go differently than anticipated. Expectant women may negotiate unexpected changes with fortitude and resilience by accepting the beauty of the unknown.

11.7 Establishing a Comfortable Birthing Setting

We talk about the importance of fostering a supportive birthing environment as we travel farther. We look at how relaxing aspects like music and aromatherapy might improve the childbirth process. Expectant women can experience safety and empowerment during childbirth by creating a soothing and supportive environment.

11.8 Postpartum Support and Planning

The celebration of the postpartum phase and the importance of postpartum preparation and support mark the chapter's conclusion. Planning for postpartum care, such as rest, good foods, and emotional support, is important, as we explore. In embracing the transforming experience of motherhood with self-love and tenderness, expectant women will discover inspiration.

The celebration of the transformational process of childbirth preparation marks the end of Chapter 11. Expectant moms may face labor with bravery, fortitude, and a sense of empowerment if they are provided with birth plans, information, coping mechanisms, and emotional support. As our trip continues, we will investigate the value of nourishing a baby and caring for the priceless life that has joined this life-changing mothering adventure.

Chapter Twelve

Newborn Care and Early Parenting: Nurturing the Precious New Life

A celebration of the birth of a priceless new life and the life-changing experience of motherhood, Chapter 12 dives into the joyful world of infant care and early parenting. We are aware that the first few weeks with a baby may be both thrilling and difficult, full of wonder and a heavy burden of duty. We examine the fundamentals of infant care in this chapter, such as eating, sleeping, changing diapers, and bonding. With love, compassion, and pleasure, new parents may set out on this transforming journey by embracing the art of caring and responsive parenting.

12.1 The Joy of Becoming a New Parent

The opening of the chapter is a celebration of the wonder and delight that come with being a new parent. We acknowledge the strong link that develops between parents and their babies as we talk about the emotional process of becoming parents. Parents who embrace the transforming potential of this new position might approach the early years with amazement and joy.

12.2 Newborn Safety and Essentials

In this part, we examine the fundamentals of infant care while highlighting the value of safety precautions. We go through the value of providing a secure sleeping environment, secure handling during diaper changes, and methods to guarantee the safety of the infant in various contexts. Parents may approach infant care with assurance and peace of mind by putting safety first.

12.3 Giving the Baby Food

We talk about the several ways to feed the infant, such as breastfeeding, formula feeding, and combination feeding, as we navigate the feeding seas. We examine the advantages of nursing for the mother and the child and provide suggestions for starting a successful breastfeeding journey. We go through the significance of responsive feeding and fostering caring feeding experiences for parents who choose formula feeding.

12.4 The Practice of Responsive Parenting and Bonding

We go into the art of bonding and responsive parenting in this part. We go through the value of snuggling, eye contact, and skin-to-skin contact in fostering the parent-child attachment. By adopting a responsive parenting approach, parents will be motivated to pay attention to their baby's indications to create security and trust.

12.5   Forming   Sound   Sleeping Patterns

As our trip continues, we examine the topic of sleep and the significance of developing sound sleeping practices. We talk about how to put your baby to sleep safely, how to make your bedroom relaxing, and how to support your baby's sleep patterns. Parents may promote peaceful sleep for both the infant and themselves by fostering appropriate sleep habits.

12.6 Care for diapers and hygiene

We go into the practical facets of diapering and hygiene care in this part. We discuss the value of ensuring good diaper cleanliness and providing solace and comfort when changing diapers. Parents will learn tips for selecting items that are soft and safe for their baby's skin.

12.7 Growing the New Family Dynamic

The chapter comes to a close with a celebration of the new family structure and the value of fostering the bonds between parents and children. We investigate the skill of striking a balance between accepting additional obligations and our family's path of development and connectedness.

The celebration of infant care and early parenthood, a magical journey of love, compassion, and pleasure, marks the conclusion of Chapter 12. New parents may set out on this transforming journey with assurance and sensitivity by embracing the fundamentals of infant care, fostering the parent-child link, and creating healthy routines. We will continue our journey by learning about the value of self-care for new parents and how to balance it with caring for the priceless child who has enriched their lives during this rewarding journey of parenting.

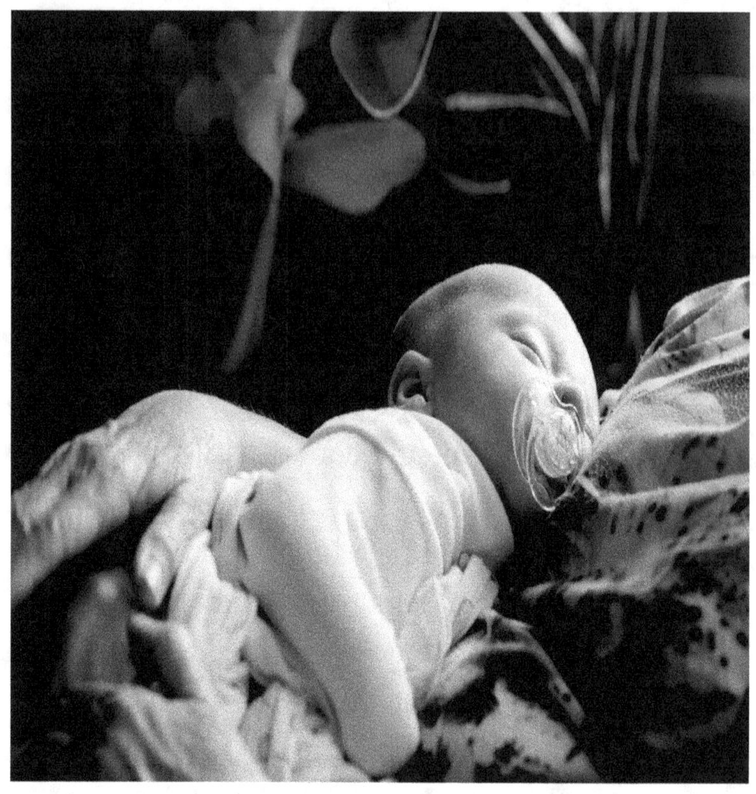

*Nutrition Solutions for Gestational Diabetes, Nausea, and Swelling*92

Chapter Thirteen

Self-Care for New Parents: Nurturing Your Well-Being During Parenthood.

With the recognition of the transformational nature of motherhood and the need of nurturing one amid the midst of the rigors of caring for a baby, Chapter 13 honors the art of self-care for new parents. We are aware that being a parent can be a very gratifying and difficult experience, and that self-care is essential to maintaining parents' physical, emotional, and mental well. This chapter looks at the usefulness of seeking help as well as the significance of self-care and practical self-nurturing techniques. New parents may travel this transforming journey with resiliency, pleasure, and a strong feeling of satisfaction if they embrace self-compassion and put their well-being first.

13.1 Accepting the Change of Becoming a Parent:

Beginning with a look at the transition to parenting, the chapter acknowledges the adjustments and emotional journey that come along with this transformational role. We talk about the benefits and difficulties of parenthood as well as the value of self-compassion. Despite the additional duties, parents may promote mental well-being by embracing this journey with compassion and tenderness.

13.2 Making self-care a priority:

In this part, we emphasize how important it is to prioritize self-care as a crucial component of parenting. We talk about how taking care of oneself is not selfish but rather a precondition for giving the infant the greatest care possible. Parents may develop a feeling of balance and well-being by identifying their needs and making time for self-nurturing.

13.3 Self-care:

We give doable methods for adding self-nurturing into everyday routines as we navigate the self-care waters. We look at the advantages of taking quick pauses for rest, participating in enjoyable pursuits, and finding quiet time for thought and renewal. Parents may preserve a sense of fulfillment among the demands of motherhood by integrating self-care into their everyday life.

13.4 Seeking Connection and Support:

We talk about the value of connecting with others throughout the early stages of motherhood in this section. We discuss the benefits of talking with other parents about your experiences, joining a support group, and asking family and friends for assistance.

Parents can find comfort and companionship on their parenting journey by building a support network.

13.5 Stress reduction and mindfulness:

We now study the advantages of mindfulness and stress-reduction practices for new parents as we continue our trip. We talk about stress-reduction techniques including deep breathing exercises, meditation, and mindfulness techniques. Parents who practice mindfulness may address problems with presence and composure.

13.6 Body Nourishment via Balanced Nutrition

The need of providing the body with a healthy diet during the postpartum period is emphasized in this section. To enhance physical well-being and energy levels, we go through the inclusion of nutrient-rich foods, hydrated liquids, and healthy meals.

13.7 Accepting Flexibility and Grace:

A celebration of grace and adaptability in the parenting experience marks the chapter's conclusion. We talk about how crucial it is to accept flaws and recognize that parenting is a learning process. Parents who are willing to let go of the drive for perfection will be able to face difficulties with resiliency and a spirit of adventure.

The celebration of new parents' self-care, a vital route to fostering well-being within the transformational experience of motherhood, marks the conclusion of Chapter 13. Parents may negotiate the rough waters of early motherhood with pleasure, contentment, and a strong feeling of connection to themselves and their priceless children by embracing self-compassion, finding help, and prioritizing their needs. On this wonderful and transformational journey of parenting, we will examine the relevance of encouraging early development and building a supportive atmosphere that promotes the newborn's growth and well-being.

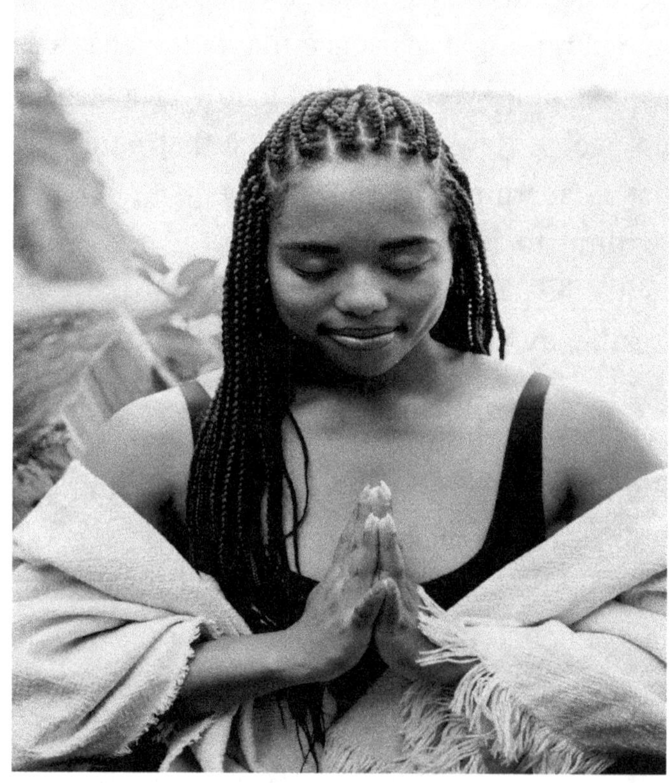

Chapter Fourteen

Fostering Early Development - Nurturing Your Newborn's Developing Mind and Body

Chapter 14 honors the amazing process of promoting infant development and acknowledges the astonishing progress and potential during the first few months of life. We are aware that a child's early growth is vital in determining how they will develop in the future and that parents are the main nurturers of this process. To assist the newborn's developing mind and body, this chapter explores the significance of responsive parenting, sensory stimulation, and creating a caring environment. Parents may help their children have a successful future by embracing this journey of learning and discovery.

14.1 Embracing Early Development's Wonders

Beginning with an examination of the miracles of early development, the chapter acknowledges the quick development and learning that takes place in the first few months of life. We talk about the value of caring parent-child relationships, sensory experiences, and brain development. Parents who embrace this journey of learning may enjoy each developmental milestone and encourage their child's growing potential.

14.2 Attachment and responsive parenting:

The importance of developing a safe and caring relationship with the newborn is emphasized as we dig into the art of responsive parenting and attachment in this part. We go through the advantages of attentive caring, reassuring cues, and responsive interactions that help the infant develop a feeling of trust and emotional stability.

14.3 Exploration and Sensory Stimulation:

We examine the significance of giving newborn children a rich sensory experience as we navigate the sensory stimulation seas. We go through the advantages of tummy time, age-appropriate toys, and stimulating experiences that enhance motor growth. Parents may encourage their child's curiosity and love of learning by promoting exploration.

14.4 Communication and Language:

In this part, we emphasize the importance of communication and language in early development. We speak about how talking, singing, and reading to a baby may improve language development and foster early literacy. Parents may encourage their baby's language development and expressive talents by engaging in an interactive conversation.

14.5 Rest and Sleep for Best Development:

We investigate the significance of sleep and rest for healthy development as our adventure continues. We go through safe sleeping habits, ways to create a restful sleeping environment, and tactics for promoting sound sleep patterns. Parents may improve their baby's general well-being and cognitive development by promoting healthy sleep.

14.6 Promoting Physical Development and Motor Skills:

In this part, we highlight the importance of supporting the newborn's physical development and motor abilities. We look at the advantages of tummy time, age-appropriate play, and encouraging activities that foster coordination and physical growth. Parents may recognize their child's accomplishments and promote their physical well-being by encouraging their development of motor skills.

14.7 Self-Expression and Emotional Control:

A celebration of emotional control and self-expression in early development marks the chapter'sTo. To support the baby's development of emotional awareness and self-regulation, we emphasize the significance of validating and acknowledging their feelings. Parents may give their children a secure and caring environment in which to explore and express their emotions by fostering their emotional well-being.

The celebration of infants' early growth, a journey of discovery, education, and love, marks the conclusion of Chapter 14. Parents may create the conditions for their child's future development and potential by practicing responsive parenting, providing sensory stimulation, and creating a supportive atmosphere. On this wonderful and transformational journey of motherhood, we will examine the value of encouraging the baby's discovery of the world, recognizing milestones, and establishing a caring and stimulating atmosphere that fosters a priceless new life.

Chapter Fifteen

Celebrating Milestones: Supporting Your Child's Growth and Development

In Chapter 15, the delightful journey of recognizing the singular and outstanding accomplishments that form a child's early years is celebrated, along with the milestones in a child's journey of growth and development. We are aware that every developmental milestone demonstrates a child's resiliency, curiosity, and potential. In this chapter, we examine the importance of recognizing accomplishments, celebrating growth, and creating a supportive atmosphere that promotes inquiry and learning. Parents who embrace this changing journey help their kids to develop with amazement and delight and treasure each milestone as a priceless memory as they travel the path of parenting.

15.1 Accepting the Growth Journey:

The first section of the chapter explores the process of growth and development, highlighting the amazing advancements made throughout a child's formative years. We talk about how the physical, cognitive, social, and emotional aspects of a child's growth are all important for their overall well-being and uniqueness. Parents may appreciate the beauty of their child's individuality and potential by embracing this journey of growth.

15.2 Fostering Milestones Through Responsive Parenting:

We go into the significance of encouraging milestones through responsive parenting in this section. We talk about how important it is to pay attention to a child's cues, support them, and explore opportunities. Parents may promote their children's ongoing learning and celebrate their triumphs by being involved and present with them.

15.3 Honoring Physical Achievers:

We examine the value of recognizing motor abilities like crawling, walking, and running as we navigate the physical milestones. We go through the advantages of age-appropriate play, outside activities, and giving kids a secure environment in which to experiment and hone their physical coordination. Parents may develop their child's sense of adventure and enjoyment of exercise by praising their physical accomplishments.

15.4 fostering cognitive milestones

Here, we emphasize the value of fostering cognitive milestones including language acquisition, analytical thinking, and early reading abilities. We talk about the importance of having dialogues, reading aloud, and developing appropriate things appropriately. Parents may encourage their children's cognitive growth and spark their interest and love of learning.

Social and emotional developmental milestones:
We investigate the value of commemorating social and emotional milestones as we continue on our journey. We talk about the value of developing connections, controlling one's emotions, and showing kindness and empathy. Parents may develop an environment of love and support that promotes emotional well-being by fostering their children's emotional intelligence.

15.6 Promoting Self-Expression and Creativity:

In this part, we highlight the importance of fostering a child's creativity and self-expression throughout their development. We talk about the importance of creativity, music, imaginative play, and chances for self-discovery. Parents may appreciate their children's particular talents and foster their individuality by encouraging creativity.

15.7 Honoring Individual Development and Resilience:

The chapter comes to a close with a celebration of a child's journey of personal development and resiliency. We talk about the value of recognizing hard work, tenacity, and the fortitude to overcome obstacles. Parents may give their kids the confidence and resilience they need to accept new experiences and learning opportunities by encouraging a growth mindset in them.

The celebration of embracing milestones, a journey of wonder, joy, and discovery, brings Chapter 15 to a close. Parents may foster their child's growth and potential with love and encouragement by supporting their child's physical, cognitive, social, and emotional milestones. On this wonderful and transforming journey of motherhood, we will examine the value of encouraging a love for lifelong learning and equipping parents to support their child's ongoing growth and development.

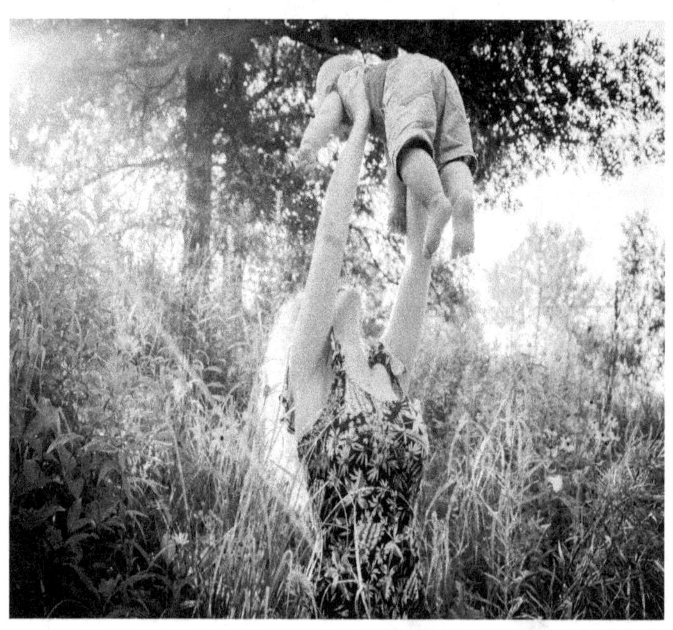

Chapter Sixteen

Pregnancy-related Diabetes

An instance of diabetes that affects how your body processes sugar (glucose) is known as gestational diabetes. It happens when the body is unable to manage blood sugar levels during pregnancy, either by producing insufficient insulin or by using it efficiently. Usually starting between the 24th and 28th week of pregnancy, gestational diabetes may go away after giving delivery. If not handled appropriately, it might have effects on both the mother and the infant.

16.1 Causes:

The placenta generates hormones during pregnancy that may affect the mother's ability to use insulin. Due to insulin resistance brought on by this hormone interference, the body requires more insulin to maintain normal blood sugar levels. Gestational diabetes arises if the body is unable to generate enough insulin to counteract this resistance.

16.2 Risk elements

Some risk factors, such as the following, make some women more susceptible to developing gestational diabetes:

1. being fat or overweight before conception.
2. having type 2 diabetes in one's family.
3. gestational diabetes from earlier plenty.
4. be over 25 years old.
5 having PCOS or polycystic ovarian syndrome.
6. A huge baby (above 9 pounds) or a child with birth abnormalities has previously been delivered.
7. having additional health issues, such as high blood pressure.

16.3 Symptoms:

Because gestational diabetes frequently has no outward signs, pregnant women should have regular prenatal screenings to identify the disease. Women may occasionally suffer increased thirst, frequent urination, or exhaustion, although these symptoms are typically related to pregnancy-related changes.

16.4 Complications:

If gestational diabetes is not well treated, both the mother and the unborn child may have complications:

1. Macrosomia: When a baby grows bigger than usual, high blood sugar levels can make labor and delivery challenging and increase the risk of birth complications.
2. Low Blood Sugar in the newborn: The newborn may have a sudden dip in blood sugar upon birth, necessitating prompt medical intervention.

3. Preterm Birth: Preterm birth is a possibility for women with gestational diabetes.

4. Preeclampsia and High Blood Pressure: The mother's risk of preeclampsia and high blood pressure during pregnancy may increase.

5. Type 2 Diabetes: Women who have gestational diabetes are more likely to go on to acquire type 2 diabetes in the future.

16.5 Management:

With a combination of a healthy diet, consistent exercise, and occasionally insulin or other drugs given by a healthcare professional, gestational diabetes can be well managed. The management of gestational diabetes requires routine blood sugar testing and adherence to an individual food plan.

In conclusion, gestational diabetes is a kind of diabetes that arises from insulin resistance during. To safeguard the health of both the mother and the unborn child, pregnant women must undergo routine prenatal screening to identify and treat the illness. Most women with gestational diabetes can have a good pregnancy and birth a healthy baby with the right care and treatment. For the duration of pregnancy, it's crucial to closely collaborate with healthcare professionals to monitor blood sugar levels and adhere to the suggested treatment schedule.

16.6 Gestational Diabetes Management

It's crucial to control gestational diabetes to protect the health of both the mother and the unborn child. Maintaining blood sugar levels within a specific range is the main objective of controlling gestation to reduce the likelihood of problems during pregnancy and delivery. Here are some essential components of gestational diabetes management:

1. Pregnant women with gestational diabetes are recommended to frequently check their blood sugar levels, often four times a day, before meals and one hour after meals. This aids in monitoring how the body reacts to food and can assist inform any necessary alterations to the diet or medical care.

2. Dietary Balance: Maintaining gestational diabetes requires adhering to a diet that is both nutritionally adequate and well-balanced. Consuming a range of nutrient-dense foods, such as whole grains, lean proteins, fruits, vegetables, and healthy fats, should be the main goal. To assist control blood sugar levels, carbohydrate consumption should be moderated and spread out evenly throughout the day.

3. Controlling portion sizes is essential for maintaining healthy blood sugar levels.

Smaller, more frequent meals can lessen the risk of post-meal blood sugar rises.

4. frequent Physical exercise: As advised by a healthcare professional, frequent physical exercise can help enhance insulin sensitivity and help manage blood sugar levels. Walking, swimming, or prenatal yoga are all safe pregnancy workouts.

5. Insulin or medication: In some situations, high blood sugar levels may persist despite lifestyle changes. In such cases, medical professionals could recommend insulin or other drugs to properly regulate blood sugar levels.

6. Regular Prenatal Checkups: It's important to get regular prenatal checkups to keep track of the baby's development and the mother's overall health. As the pregnancy develops, medical professionals will monitor blood sugar levels and modify the treatment strategy as necessary.

7. Monitoring Blood Pressure: It's important to keep an eye on your blood pressure since gestational diabetes raises your risk of preeclampsia and high blood pressure throughout pregnancy.

8. Self-care and stress reduction: It's important to take care of yourself while you're pregnant. Blood sugar levels can be impacted by stress, therefore it's important to find strategies to decompress and unwind for general well-being.

9. Education and Support: Attending seminars on gestational diabetes and asking for assistance from medical professionals, nutritionists, and other pregnant people with the condition can be beneficial. Sharing stories and learning more about the illness may be incredibly insightful and motivating.

It's crucial to keep in mind that each woman's experience with gestational diabetes is distinct, and the care strategy may change depending on her requirements.

A good perspective, commitment to the recommended treatment plan, and open contact with healthcare professionals are essential components of treating gestational diabetes successfully.

Most women with gestational diabetes can have a good pregnancy and birth a healthy baby with careful treatment. Blood sugar levels often return to normal following delivery. However, type 2 diabetes in later life is more likely to strike women with gestation. To monitor long-term health and implement the appropriate preventative measures, constant follow-up with healthcare specialists is needed.

Nutrition Solutions for Gestational Diabetes, Nausea, and Swelling

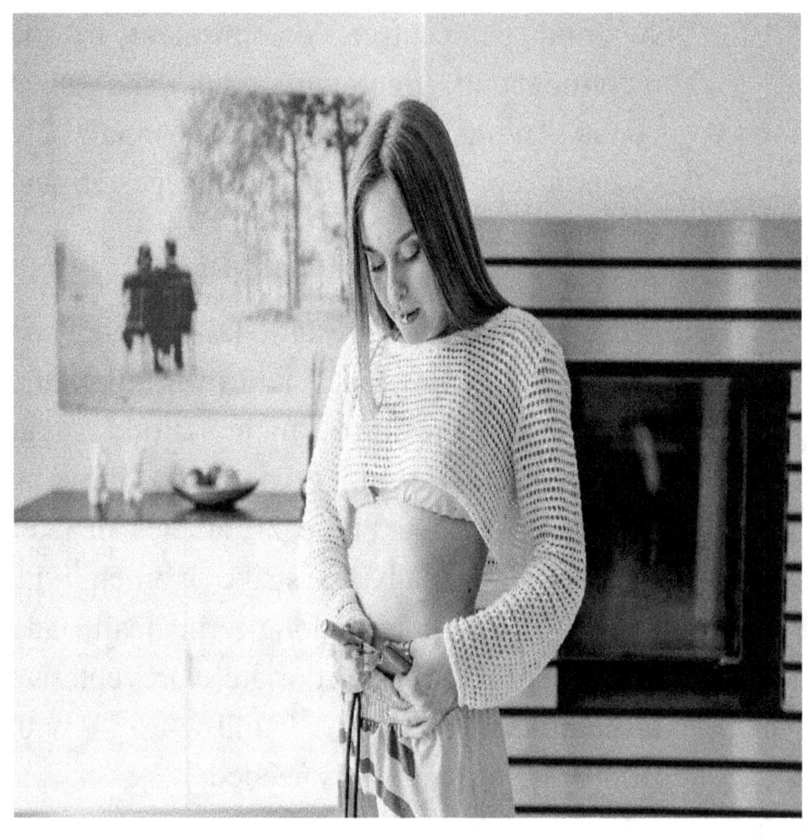

Nutrition Solutions for Gestational Diabetes, Nausea, and Swelling120

Conclusion

The transforming journey of motherhood, where love, wonder, and development merge to produce a deep and gratifying experience, is celebrated as we approach the book's last chapter. A voyage of discovery, education, and empowerment, "Addressing Common Concerns: Nutrition Solutions for Gestational Diabetes, Nausea, and Swelling" helps expecting moms and new parents navigate the harsh waters of pregnancy and early parenting.

We have covered important subjects including controlling gestational diabetes, dealing with typical pregnancy worries, nourishing the developing mind and body of the infant, and promoting early developmental milestones throughout this book. Practical advice, insightful commentary, and encouraging direction are offered in each chapter to help parents on their transforming journey.

We now understand the significance of a balanced diet that nourishes both the mother and the unborn child throughout pregnancy. We have looked at useful solutions that support health and well-being, from controlling gestational diabetes to reducing nausea and swelling.

In light of the rigors of motherhood, the art of self-care has been promoted, urging parents to take care of their physical, emotional, and mental health. Parents may successfully navigate the parenting waters by prioritizing self-compassion and seeking help.

We are now aware of the marvels of early development, and we see each milestone as a symbol of a child's development and potential. Parents may watch their child's exploration and learning journey with wonder and love by providing responsive parenting, caring settings, and supporting interactions.

Let us keep in mind that motherhood is a transformational journey of development, learning, and love as we say goodbye to this adventure. Parents may handle the trials and rewards of raising a family with grace and contentment by embracing the individuality and potential of each kid.

May you use this book as a compass and a travel companion on your parenting journey, leading you through the highs and lows with knowledge, encouragement, and To. To build treasured experiences that will forever add to the fabric of your family's tale, embrace the art of compassionate care as you proceed along your path.

May you experience love, joy, and the wonder of watching a priceless life develop in front of your own eyes on your journey. I'm wishing you well as you go out on the transformational and wonderful journey that is motherhood. Happy travels!